Juicing Recipes For Cancer Patients

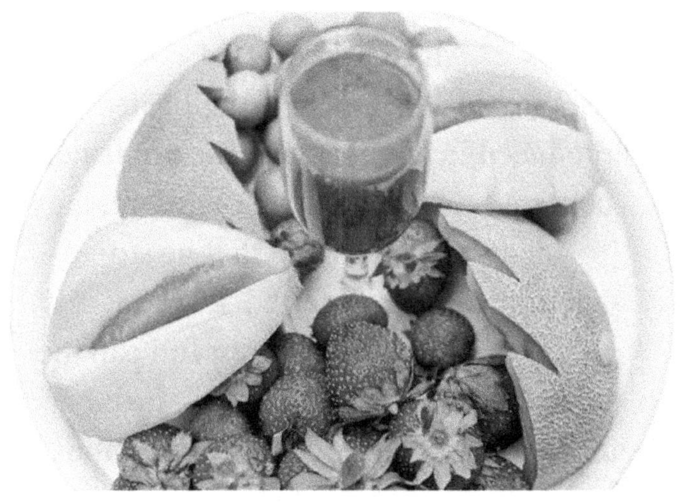

35 Nutritious Juices to prevent, manage and fight cancer

Joshua S. Gray

For more information or help feel free to contact me at:
joshuagrayhelpdesk@gmail.com

Thank you for purchasing this book.

Table of Contents

CLICK HERE TO GET CANCER FIGHTING RECIPES FOR NEWLY DIAGNOSED

Introduction

Jane's journey to overcoming cancer was filled with determination, hope, and a transformative approach to nutrition.

When diagnosed with cancer, she sought ways to optimize her well-being during treatment, and it was through the power of juicing recipes that she discovered a remarkable ally in her healing process.

Recognizing the potential of fruits, vegetables, and herbs, Jane embraced a juicing regimen tailored to her unique needs. By extracting the pure essence of vibrant produce, she unlocked a wealth of vital nutrients, antioxidants, and phytochemicals in every invigorating glass.

These liquid elixirs not only nourished her body but also revitalized her spirit.

In this collection of juicing recipes for cancer patients, we embark on a journey inspired by Jane's transformative experience.

From refreshing citrus blends to vibrant green concoctions, each recipe is thoughtfully crafted to provide a symphony of flavors, while delivering a concentrated dose of essential nutrients.

Join me as we explore the rejuvenating power of juicing, and discover how these recipes can nourish and support the well-being of cancer patients on their own unique paths to healing.

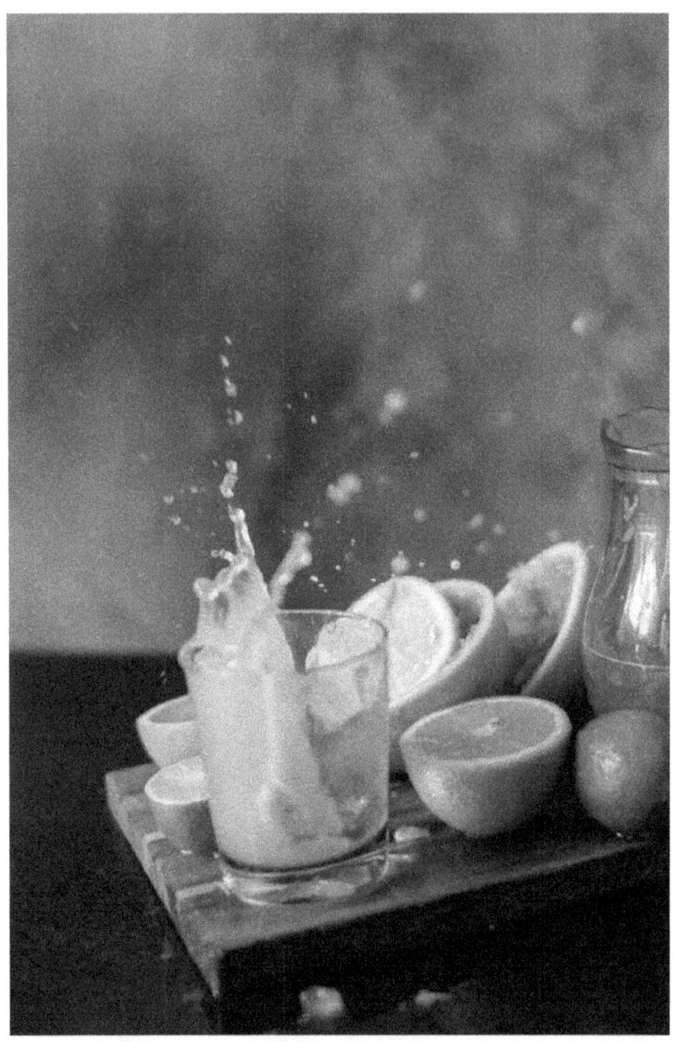

Importance of Juicing for Cancer Patients

Juicing can hold significant importance for cancer patients as it offers several potential benefits to support their overall well-being during and after treatment. Here are some key reasons why juicing is valuable for cancer patients:

1.   **Nutrient Density:** Juicing allows for the extraction of concentrated nutrients from fruits, vegetables, and herbs. It provides a convenient and easily digestible way to consume a wide range of vitamins, minerals, antioxidants, and phytochemicals that are essential for cellular repair, immune function, and overall health. This nutrient

density helps support the body's healing processes and provides a boost of essential nutrients, especially if appetite or digestion is affected by cancer treatments.

2.   **Hydration:**   Staying   properly hydrated is crucial for cancer patients. Juicing can contribute to their hydration status, as many fruits and vegetables have high water content. Juices can provide a refreshing and hydrating source of fluids, especially when combined with water-rich ingredients like cucumber, watermelon, or citrus fruits.

3.   **Digestive Comfort:** Some cancer treatments can lead to digestive discomfort, such as nausea, vomiting, or mouth sores, which may make it challenging to consume

whole foods. Juicing can offer a solution by providing easily digestible nutrients in a gentle form. It allows patients to obtain essential vitamins and minerals without putting additional strain on their digestive system.

4. **Antioxidant and Anti-inflammatory Support:** Juices derived from colorful fruits and vegetables are rich in antioxidants and anti-inflammatory compounds. These properties can help combat oxidative stress, reduce inflammation, and support the body's defense mechanisms against cancer cells. Antioxidants can also aid in protecting healthy cells from damage caused by treatments like chemotherapy or radiation therapy.

5. **Boosting Immune Function:** Cancer and its treatments can weaken the immune system. Juices packed with immune-boosting nutrients, such as vitamin C, beta-carotene, and zinc, can strengthen the immune system and enhance its ability to fight infections, thereby supporting overall health and reducing the risk of complications.

6.   Palatability and Variety: Juicing offers cancer patients the opportunity to enjoy a wide range of flavors and tastes, even if they have altered taste perceptions due to treatments. By combining different fruits, vegetables, and herbs, patients can experiment with flavors and textures, making their nutritional intake more enjoyable and diverse.

While juicing can provide valuable benefits for cancer patients, it's essential to note that it should not replace a well-balanced diet or medical treatments. Juices should be used as a supplement to a healthy eating plan and consumed in moderation.

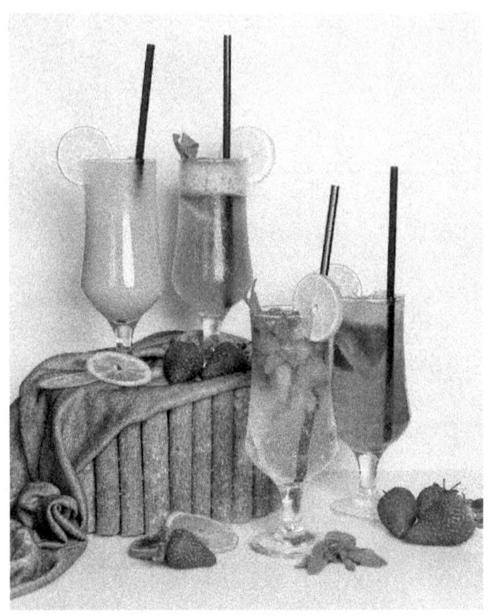

Juicing Recipes For Cancer Patients

Here are 35 juicing recipes and their preparation instructions that are suitable for cancer patients:

1. Green Goddess

Ingredients:

- 1 cup spinach

- 1 cup kale

- 1 cucumber

- 1 green apple

- 1 lemon (juiced)

Preparation:

Run all the ingredients through a juicer. Stir well and serve chilled.

2.   Berry Blast

Ingredients:

- 1 cup mixed strawberries, or blueberries, or raspberries
- 1 cup spinach
- 1 banana
- 1 cup almond milk

Preparation:

Blend all the ingredients together until smooth. Adjust the consistency by adding more almond milk if desired.

3.   Carrot Ginger Zing

Ingredients:

- 3 carrots

- 1-inch piece of fresh ginger

- 1 apple

- 1 lemon (juiced)

Preparation:

Juice the carrots, ginger, apple, and lemon. Stir well and enjoy the zesty flavor.

4.   Citrus Sunrise

Ingredients:

- 2 oranges

- 1 grapefruit

- 1 lemon

- 1-inch piece of turmeric (optional)

Preparation:

Juice the oranges, grapefruit, lemon, and turmeric. Pour into a glass and savor the refreshing citrus flavors.

5. Beetroot Booster

Ingredients:

- 1 beetroot
- 2 carrots
- 1 apple
- 1-inch piece of ginger
- 1 lemon (juiced)

Preparation:

Run all the ingredients through a juicer. Mix well and serve chilled for a nutrient-packed boost.

6.   Tropical Paradise

Ingredients:

- 1 cup pineapple chunks

- 1 banana

- 1 cup spinach

- 1 cup coconut water

Preparation:

Blend all the ingredients until smooth. Add more coconut water if needed to achieve the desired consistency.

7.　Healing Turmeric Blend

Ingredients:

- 2 carrots

- 1 apple

- 1-inch piece of turmeric

- 1 lemon (juiced)

- Pinch of black pepper

Preparation:

Juice the carrots, apple, turmeric, and lemon. Sprinkle a pinch of black pepper and stir well.

8.   Refreshing   Minty Watermelon

Ingredients:

- 2 cups watermelon chunks

- 1 handful fresh mint leaves

- 1 lime (juiced)

Preparation:

Blend the watermelon and mint leaves until smooth. Stir and serve.

9.   Immune Booster

Ingredients:

- 1 orange

- 1 carrot

- 1-inch piece of ginger

- 1 small beetroot

- 1 lemon (juiced)

Preparation:

Juice the orange, carrot, ginger, beetroot, and lemon. Mix well and enjoy the immune-boosting goodness.

10. Cucumber Cooler

Ingredients:

- 1 cucumber
- 1 cup honeydew melon chunks
- 1 lime (juiced)
- Handful of fresh basil leaves

Preparation:

Blend the cucumber, honeydew melon, lime juice, and basil until smooth. Strain if desired and serve chilled.

11.   Kale Power Punch

Ingredients:

- 2 cups kale

- 1 green apple

- 1 cucumber

- 1 lemon (juiced)

- 1-inch piece of ginger

Preparation:

Run all the ingredients through a juicer. Stir well and enjoy the invigorating green goodness.

12.   Mango Tango

Ingredients:

- 1 ripe mango

- 1 banana

- 1 cup spinach

- 1 cup coconut water

Preparation:

Blend all the ingredients until smooth. Add more coconut water if necessary.

13. Antioxidant Elixir

Ingredients:

- 1 cup blueberries

- 1 cup strawberries

- 1 cup raspberries

- 1 cup spinach

- 1 lemon (juiced)

Preparation:

Juice the blueberries, strawberries, raspberries, spinach, and lemon. Mix well and savor the antioxidant-rich elixir.

14. Zesty Carrot Apple

Ingredients:

- 3 carrots

- 2 apples

- 1 lemon (juiced)

- 1-inch piece of ginger

Preparation:

Juice the carrots, apples, ginger, and lemon.
Stir well and enjoy the zingy combination.

15. Pineapple Mint Delight

Ingredients:

- 1 cup pineapple chunks

- Handful of fresh mint leaves

- 1 cucumber

- 1 lime (juiced)

Preparation:

Blend the pineapple, mint leaves, cucumber, and lime juice until smooth.

16. Immune-Boosting Citrus

Ingredients:

- 2 oranges

- 1 grapefruit

- 2 lemons (juiced)

- 1-inch piece of turmeric

- Pinch of cayenne pepper (optional for a kick)

Preparation:

Juice the oranges, grapefruit, lemons, and turmeric. You can add a little cayenne pepper. Stir well and enjoy the immune-boosting goodness.

17. Green Detoxifier

Ingredients:

- 2 cups spinach

- 1 cucumber

- 1 green apple

- 1 lemon (juiced)

- Handful of fresh parsley

Preparation:

Run all the ingredients through a juicer. Mix well and savor the cleansing properties of this green detoxifier.

18. Purple Powerhouse

Ingredients:

- 1 cup purple grapes

- 1 cup blueberries

- 1 cup spinach

- 1 banana

- 1 cup almond milk

Preparation:

Blend all the ingredients until smooth. Almond milk can be added.

19. Ginger Lemon Elixir

Ingredients:

- 2 lemons (juiced)

- 1-inch piece of ginger

- 1 tablespoon honey (optional)

- Pinch of turmeric (optional)

Preparation:

Juice the lemons and ginger. Add honey and turmeric if desired, and stir well to combine. Serve chilled.

20. Watermelon Cucumber Refresher

Ingredients:

- 2 cups watermelon chunks
- 1 cucumber
- Handful of fresh mint leaves
- 1 lime (juiced)

Preparation:

Blend the watermelon, cucumber, mint leaves, and lime juice until smooth. Serve over ice for a refreshing and hydrating drink.

21. Citrus Beet Cleanse

Ingredients:

- 1 beetroot

- 2 oranges

- 1 lemon (juiced)

- 1-inch piece of ginger

Preparation:

Juice the beetroot, oranges, lemon, and ginger. Stir well and enjoy the cleansing and detoxifying properties.

22. Kale Pineapple Fusion

Ingredients:

- 2 cups kale

- 1 cup pineapple chunks

- 1 green apple

- 1 lemon (juiced)

Preparation:

Run all the ingredients through a juicer. Stir well and savor the tropical fusion of flavors.

23. Carrot Turmeric Elixir

Ingredients:

- 3 carrots

- 1 orange

- 1-inch piece of turmeric

- 1 lemon (juiced)

Preparation:

Juice the carrots, orange, turmeric, and lemon. Stir well and enjoy the vibrant color and immune-boosting properties.

24. Mango Spinach Surprise

Ingredients:

- 1 ripe Mango

- 2 cups spinach

- 1 banana

- 1 cup coconut water

Preparation:

Blend all the ingredients until smooth. Add more coconut water if needed to reach the desired consistency.

25. Raspberry Mint Lemonade

Ingredients:

- 1 cup raspberries

- Handful of fresh mint leaves

- 2 lemons (juiced)

- 1 tablespoon honey (optional)

Preparation:

Blend the raspberries, mint leaves, lemon juice, and honey (if using) until smooth.

26. Pineapple Kale Energizer

Ingredients:

- 1 cup pineapple chunks

- 2 cups kale

- 1 green apple

- 1 lemon (juiced)

Preparation:

Run all the ingredients through a juicer. Stir well and enjoy the energizing blend.

27. Carrot Orange Splash

Ingredients:

- 3 carrots

- 2 oranges

- 1-inch piece of ginger

- 1 lemon (juiced)

Juice the carrots, oranges, ginger, and lemon. Mix well and savor the vibrant splash of citrus.

28. Cucumber Kiwi Refresher

Ingredients:

- 1 cucumber

- 2 kiwis

- Handful of fresh mint leaves

- 1 lime (juiced)

Preparation:

Cucumber, kiwi fruit, mint leaves, and lime juice are mixed together in a blender until smooth. Serve chilled for a refreshing pick-me-up.

29. Berry Green Dream

Ingredients:

- 1 cup mixed strawberries, or blueberries, or raspberries.
- 2 cups spinach
- 1 banana
- 1 cup almond milk

Preparation:

Blend all the ingredients until smooth. Adjust the consistency with more almond milk if desired.

30. Ginger Pear Bliss

Ingredients:

- 2 pears

- 1-inch piece of ginger

- 1 lemon (juiced)

- 1 tablespoon honey (optional)

Preparation:

Juice the pears and ginger. Stir in the lemon juice and honey (if desired) for a blissful and soothing drink.

31. Golden Glow Turmeric Blend

Ingredients:

- 2 carrots

- 1 orange

- 1-inch piece of turmeric

- 1 lemon (juiced)

- Pinch of black pepper

Preparation:

Juice the carrots, orange, turmeric, and lemon. Add a pinch of black pepper and stir well to combine the flavors.

32.   Green Apple Detox

Ingredients:

- 2 green apples

- 2 cups spinach

- 1 cucumber

- 1 lemon (juiced)

- Handful of fresh parsley

Preparation:

Run all the ingredients through a juicer. Mix well and enjoy the detoxifying benefits of this green apple concoction.

33. Blueberry Beet Blast

Ingredients:

- 1 cup blueberries

- 1 small beetroot

- 1 banana

- 1 cup almond milk

- 1 tablespoon chia seeds (optional)

Preparation:

Blend all the ingredients until smooth. Add chia seeds for added nutrition if desired.

34. Citrus Carrot Ginger

Ingredients:

- 3 carrots

- 2 oranges

- 1 lemon (juiced)

- 1-inch piece of ginger

Preparation:

Juice the carrots, oranges, lemon, and ginger. Stir well and enjoy the invigorating blend of citrus and ginger.

35. Mango Coconut Delight

Ingredients:

- 1 ripe mango

- 1 cup coconut water

- 1 lime (juiced)

- Handful of fresh mint leaves

Preparation:

Blend the mango, coconut water, lime juice, and mint leaves until smooth. Serve chilled for a tropical and refreshing treat.

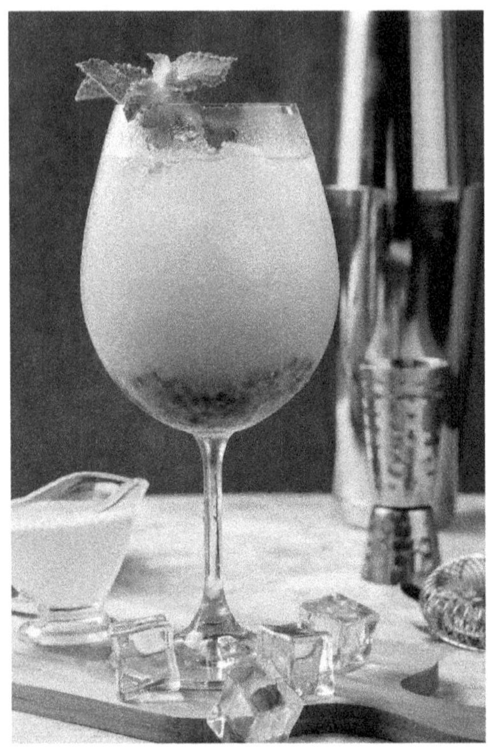

21-Day Juicing Plan

Here's a 21-day juicing plan for cancer patients. Each day includes a different juicing recipe to provide variety and ensure a range of nutrients.

Day 1:

Green Goddess

Ingredients:

- 1 cup spinach

- 1 cup kale

- 1 cucumber

- 1 green apple

- 1 lemon (juiced)

Day 2:

Carrot Ginger Zing

Ingredients:

- 3 carrots

- 1-inch piece of fresh ginger

- 1 apple

- 1 lemon (juiced)

Day 3:

Berry Blast

Ingredients:

- 1 cup mixed strawberries, or blueberries, or raspberries.

- 1 cup spinach

- 1 banana

- 1 cup almond milk

Day 4:

Citrus Sunrise

Ingredients:

- 2 oranges

- 1 grapefruit

- 1 lemon

- 1-inch piece of turmeric (optional)

Day 5:

Beetroot Booster

Ingredients:

- 1 beetroot

- 2 carrots

- 1 apple

- 1-inch piece of ginger

- 1 lemon (juiced)

Day 6:

Tropical Paradise

Ingredients:

- 1 cup pineapple chunks

- 1 banana

- 1 cup spinach

- 1 cup coconut water

Day 7:

Healing Turmeric Blend

Ingredients:

- 2 carrots

- 1 apple

- 1-inch piece of turmeric

- 1 lemon (juiced)

- Pinch of black pepper

Day 8:

Refreshing Minty Watermelon

Ingredients:

- 2 cups watermelon chunks

- 1 handful fresh mint leaves

- 1 lime (juiced)

Day 9:

Immune Booster

Ingredients:

- 1 orange

- 1 carrot

- 1-inch piece of ginger

- 1 small beetroot

- 1 lemon (juiced)

Day 10:

Cucumber Cooler

Ingredients:

- 1 cucumber

- 1 cup honeydew melon chunks

- 1 lime (juiced)

- Handful of fresh basil leaves

Day 11:

Kale Power Punch

Ingredients:

- 2 cups kale

- 1 green apple

- 1 cucumber

- 1 lemon (juiced)

- 1-inch piece of ginger

Day 12:

Mango Tango

Ingredients:

- 1 ripe mango

- 1 banana

- 1 cup spinach

- 1 cup coconut water

Day 13:

Antioxidant Elixir

Ingredients:

- 1 cup blueberries

- 1 cup strawberries

- 1 cup raspberries

- 1 cup spinach

- 1 lemon (juiced)

Day 14:

Zesty Carrot Apple

Ingredients:

- 3 carrots

- 2 apples

- 1 lemon (juiced)

- 1-inch piece of ginger

Day 15:

Pineapple Mint Delight

Ingredients:

- 1 cup pineapple chunks

- Handful of fresh mint leaves

- 1 lime (juiced)

Day 16:

Immune-Boosting Citrus

Ingredients:

- 2 oranges

- 1 grapefruit

- 2 lemons (juiced)

- 1-inch piece of turmeric

- Pinch of cayenne pepper (optional for a kick)

Day 17:

Green Detoxifier

Ingredients:

- 2 cups spinach

- 1 cucumber

- 1 green apple

- 1 lemon (juiced)

- Handful of fresh parsley

Day 18:

Purple Powerhouse

Ingredients:

- 1 cup purple grapes

- 1 cup blueberries

- 1 cup spinach

- 1 banana

- 1 cup almond milk

Day 19:

Ginger Lemon Elixir

Ingredients:

- 2 lemons (juiced)

- 1-inch piece of ginger

- 1 tablespoon honey (optional)

- Pinch of turmeric (optional)

Day 20:

Watermelon Cucumber Refresher

Ingredients:

- 2 cups watermelon chunks

- 1 cucumber

- Handful of fresh mint leaves

- 1 lime (juiced)

Day 21:

Citrus Beet Cleanse

Ingredients:

- 1 beetroot

- 2 oranges

- 1 lemon (juiced)

- 1-inch piece of ginger

Feel free to repeat the recipes from Day 1 onwards after completing the 21-day plan.

Remember to listen to your body's needs and make adjustments as necessary. Juicing can be a healthy addition to your overall diet, but it's important to consume a balanced and varied diet to meet all your nutritional requirements.

Conclusion

In conclusion, juicing can be a valuable addition to the dietary regimen of cancer patients. The juicing recipes specifically designed for cancer patients offer a wide range of benefits. They provide a concentrated dose of essential nutrients, vitamins, and minerals that can support the body's natural healing processes, boost the immune system, and enhance overall well-being.

The recipes mentioned in this book offer a variety of flavors and combinations to suit individual preferences while ensuring a diverse range of nutrients. From antioxidant-rich elixirs to detoxifying blends, each recipe serves a specific purpose in promoting health and vitality.

It is crucial for cancer patients to consult with healthcare professionals or registered dietitians to ensure that these juicing recipes align with their specific dietary needs and treatment plans. Additionally, it is important to remember that juicing should not replace a well-rounded diet but should complement it.

By incorporating these juicing recipes into their lifestyle, cancer patients can nourish their bodies, support their immune systems, and potentially experience the benefits of improved energy, enhanced digestion, and overall well-being. Juicing can be a valuable tool on their journey towards better health and vitality.

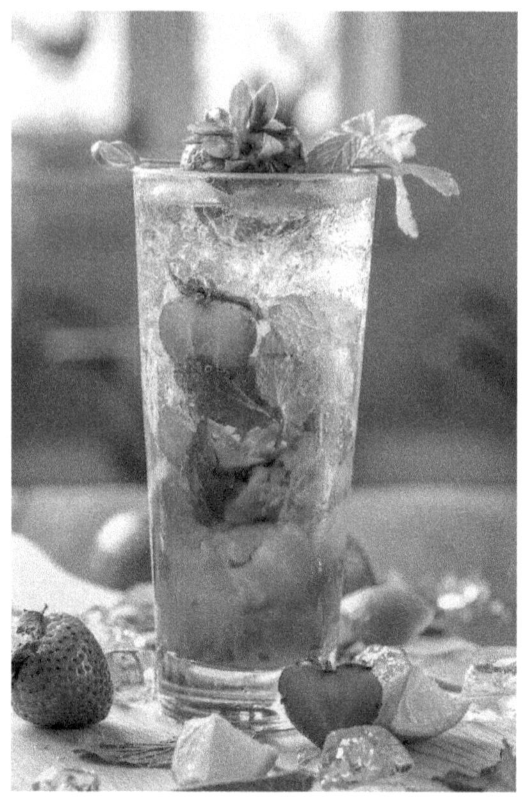

Thank You For Reading!